THE GALLBLADDER DIET COOKBOOK FOR BEGINNERS

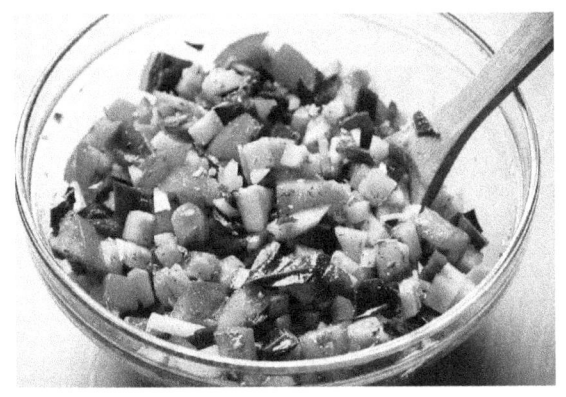

DR. JESSICA SMITH

Copyright © 2024 by DR. JESSICA SMITH

All rights reserved.

No part of this book may be reproduced, stored in a retrieval system, or transmitted, in any form or by any means, electronic, mechanical, photocopying, recording, or otherwise, without prior written permission from the publisher, except for brief quotations embodied in critical articles or reviews.

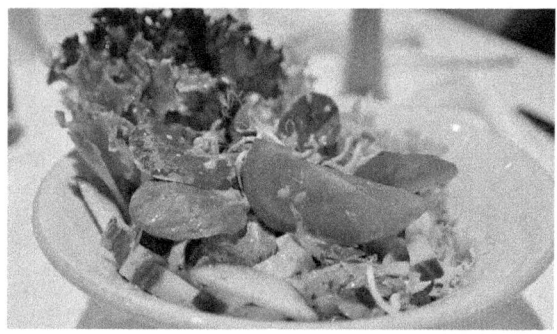

TABLE OF CONTENTS

CHAPTER ONE 7

How to Use this Cookbook 7

Understanding Gallbladder Diet for Beginners .. 9

Benefits of Gallbladder Diet For Beginners 10

Guidelines for Gallbladder Diet for Beginners 12

CHAPTER TWO 15

Gallbladder Diet Breakfast Recipes for Beginners
.... 15

1: Veggie Omelette 15

2: Greek Yogurt Parfait 16

3: Banana Oatmeal 18

4: Avocado Toast 19

5: Spinach and Feta Egg Muffins 21

6: Chia Seed Pudding 22

7: Cottage Cheese Pancakes 24

8: Quinoa Breakfast Bowl 25

9: Apple Cinnamon Overnight Oats 27

10: Sweet Potato Breakfast Hash 29

Gallbladder Diet Lunch Recipes for Beginners 31

1: Grilled Lemon Herb Chicken Salad 31

2: Quinoa and Black Bean Stuffed Bell Peppers 33

3: Baked Salmon with Roasted Vegetables 35

4: Lentil and Vegetable Soup 37

5: Turkey and Avocado Wrap 39

6: Quinoa Salad with Lemon Herb Dressing....41

7: Chickpea Salad Sandwich 42

8: Zucchini Noodles with Pesto and Cherry Tomatoes 44

9: Tuna Salad Lettuce Wraps 46

10: Veggie Stir-Fry with Brown Rice 48

Gallbladder Diet Dinner Recipes for Beginners 50

1: Baked Lemon Herb Salmon 50

2: Quinoa and Vegetable Stir-Fry 52

3: Roasted Chicken with Sweet Potatoes and Broccoli 54

4: Lentil and Vegetable Soup 56

5: Turkey and Vegetable Skillet 58

6: Stuffed Bell Peppers with Quinoa and Black Beans 60

7: Grilled Lemon Herb Chicken with Steamed Vegetables 62

8: Baked Cod with Roasted Asparagus 64

9: Vegetarian Lentil Soup 66

10: Baked Chicken and Vegetable Sheet Pan Dinner 68

Gallbladder Diet Snacks Recipes for Beginners 70

1: Greek Yogurt Parfait with Berries 70

2: Hummus and Vegetable Crudité Platter 71

3: Apple Slices with Almond Butter 73

4: Cottage Cheese and Pineapple Kabobs 74

5: Avocado Toast with Tomato 75

6: Rice Cake with Almond Butter and Banana. 76

7: Veggie Sticks with Yogurt Dip 78

8: Almond and Berry Smoothie 79

9: Baked Sweet Potato Chips 80

10: Cottage Cheese and Fruit Bowl 82

CONCLUSION 84

CHAPTER ONE

How to Use this Cookbook

Understand Your Diet Goals: Start by understanding why you're following a gallbladder diet. Typically, it's to reduce symptoms like bloating, gas, and pain caused by gallstones or other gallbladder issues.

Educate Yourself: Learn which foods trigger your symptoms and which are safe to eat. Common trigger foods include high-fat, greasy, spicy, and processed foods.

Consult a Healthcare Professional: Before making any significant dietary changes, it's essential to consult your healthcare provider or a registered dietitian. They can provide personalized advice based on your specific condition and needs.

Focus on Low-Fat Foods: The cornerstone of a gallbladder diet is low-fat foods. Choose lean proteins like chicken, turkey, fish, and legumes, and opt for low-fat dairy products.

Incorporate High-Fiber Foods: High-fiber foods can help regulate digestion and prevent constipation, which is beneficial for gallbladder health. Include plenty of fruits, vegetables, whole grains, and legumes in your meals.

Stay Hydrated: Drink plenty of water throughout the day to help maintain good digestion and prevent dehydration, which can worsen gallbladder symptoms.

Limit Trigger Foods: Avoid or limit foods that commonly trigger gallbladder symptoms, such as fatty meats, fried foods, processed snacks, spicy foods, and high-fat dairy products.

Practice Portion Control: Even healthy foods can trigger symptoms if consumed in large quantities. Be mindful of portion sizes, especially with high-fat or high-fiber foods.

Eat Regular Meals: Establish a regular eating schedule and try to eat smaller, more frequent meals rather than large, heavy meals. This can help prevent overloading your digestive system and minimize symptoms.

Monitor Your Symptoms: Pay attention to how your body responds to different foods and adjust your diet accordingly. Keeping a food diary can help you identify trigger foods and track your progress over time.

Understanding Gallbladder Diet for Beginners

Understanding the gallbladder diet for beginners is crucial for managing symptoms and promoting gallbladder health.

This dietary approach focuses on reducing the consumption of foods that can trigger discomfort or exacerbate gallbladder issues, such as gallstones or inflammation.

The primary goal of the gallbladder diet is to minimize the workload on the gallbladder by limiting the intake of high-fat, greasy, spicy, and processed foods.

These foods can lead to the production of excessive bile, which may exacerbate symptoms like pain, bloating, gas, and indigestion.

Beginners should familiarize themselves with the types of foods that are considered safe and beneficial for gallbladder health.

These include lean proteins like poultry, fish, and legumes, as well as low-fat dairy products. High-fiber foods such as fruits, vegetables, whole grains, and legumes are also encouraged as they promote regular digestion and prevent constipation.

Portion control is another essential aspect of the gallbladder diet. Even healthy foods can trigger symptoms if consumed in large quantities, so beginners should pay attention to serving sizes and avoid overeating.

Staying hydrated by drinking plenty of water throughout the day can help maintain good digestion and prevent dehydration, which can worsen gallbladder symptoms.

Benefits of Gallbladder Diet For Beginners

The benefits of following a gallbladder diet for beginners are numerous and can significantly improve overall health and well-being.

Here are some key advantages:

Symptom Management: One of the primary benefits of the gallbladder diet is the effective management of symptoms associated with gallbladder issues, such as pain, bloating, gas, and indigestion.

Prevention of Complications: Following a gallbladder diet can help prevent complications such as gallstones or inflammation of the gallbladder (cholecystitis). By reducing the workload on the gallbladder and promoting healthy digestion, beginners can lower their risk of developing these issues.

Improved Digestive Health: The gallbladder diet emphasizes the consumption of high-fiber foods, lean proteins, and low-fat options, which can promote regular digestion and prevent constipation. This leads to better overall digestive health and reduces the likelihood of experiencing gastrointestinal problems.

Weight Management: Since the gallbladder diet encourages the consumption of nutritious, whole foods while limiting high-fat and processed options, it can support weight management efforts.

By making healthier food choices and practicing portion control, beginners can achieve and maintain a healthy weight, which is essential for gallbladder health.

The gallbladder diet offers beginners a holistic approach to managing symptoms, preventing complications, and promoting overall health and well-being. With proper guidance and adherence to dietary principles, individuals can experience significant benefits and enjoy a better quality of life.

Guidelines for Gallbladder Diet for Beginners

For beginners embarking on a gallbladder diet journey, adhering to specific guidelines is crucial for managing symptoms effectively and promoting gallbladder health. Here's a comprehensive set of guidelines:

Consult Healthcare Professionals: Seek guidance from healthcare providers or registered dietitians to develop a personalized gallbladder diet plan tailored to your individual needs and condition.

Educate Yourself: Learn about foods that trigger gallbladder symptoms and those that are safe to consume. This knowledge forms the foundation of your dietary choices.

Focus on Low-Fat Options: Prioritize low-fat foods, including lean proteins like chicken, turkey, and fish, and opt for low-fat dairy products to reduce the strain on your gallbladder.

Incorporate High-Fiber Foods: Integrate fiber-rich foods such as fruits, vegetables, whole grains, and legumes into your diet to support digestion and prevent constipation.

Stay Hydrated: Drink an adequate amount of water throughout the day to maintain hydration and support optimal digestion, which can alleviate gallbladder symptoms.

Limit Trigger Foods: Avoid or minimize consumption of trigger foods such as fatty meats, fried foods, processed snacks, spicy dishes, and high-fat dairy products to prevent symptom flare-ups.

Practice Portion Control: Monitor portion sizes to prevent overeating, even with healthy foods, as large meals can overload your digestive system and exacerbate symptoms.

Eat Regularly: Establish a consistent eating schedule with smaller, more frequent meals to regulate digestion and prevent digestive discomfort.

Monitor Symptoms: Keep track of how your body responds to different foods and adjust your diet accordingly. A food diary can help identify trigger foods and track progress.

Be Patient and Persistent: Understand that dietary changes take time to yield noticeable results. Stay committed to your gallbladder diet plan and be patient as you work towards better symptom management and improved gallbladder health.

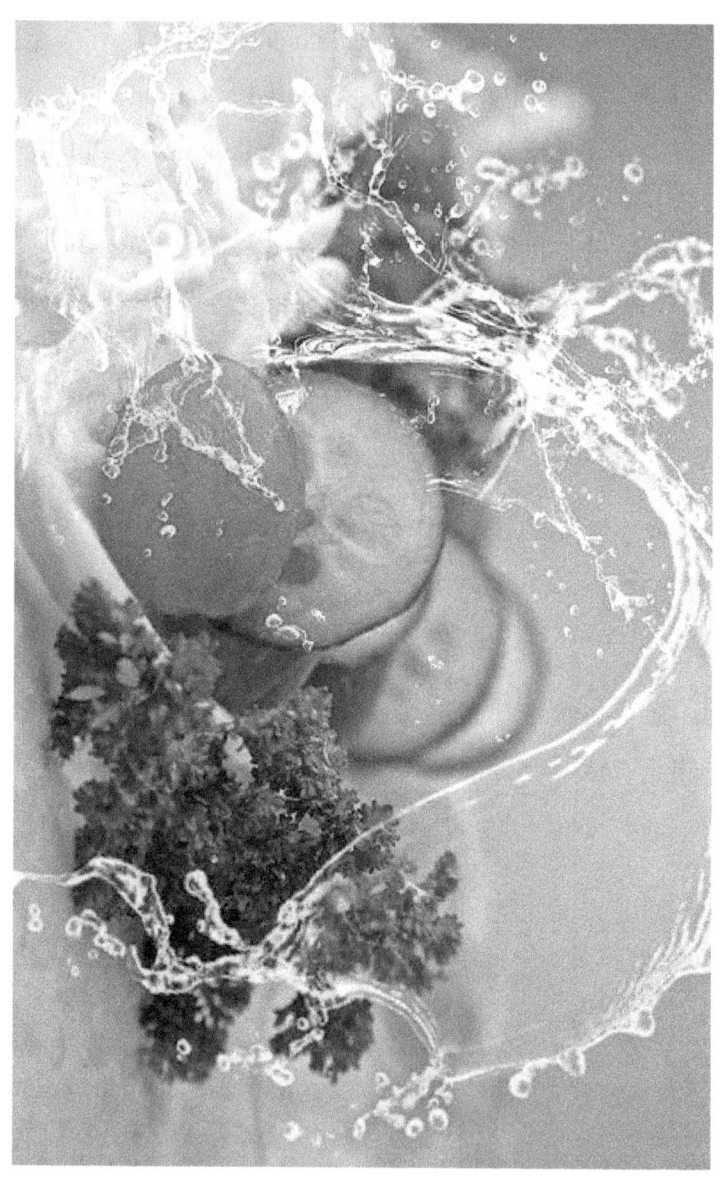

CHAPTER TWO

Gallbladder Diet Breakfast Recipes for Beginners

1: Veggie Omelette

Ingredients:

- 2 eggs
- 1/4 cup chopped bell peppers (any color)
- 1/4 cup chopped tomatoes
- 1/4 cup chopped spinach
- Salt and pepper to taste
- 1 teaspoon olive oil

Instructions:

- Heat olive oil in a non-stick skillet over medium heat.
- In a bowl, whisk together eggs, salt, and pepper.
- Pour the egg mixture into the skillet and let it cook for a minute until the edges start to set.
- Sprinkle chopped bell peppers, tomatoes, and spinach evenly over the eggs.

- Cook for another 2-3 minutes until the bottom is golden brown and the vegetables are slightly softened.
- Fold the omelette in half using a spatula and cook for another minute until the eggs are fully cooked through.
- Transfer the omelette to a plate and serve hot.

Health Benefits:

- This veggie omelette is high in protein from the eggs and packed with vitamins and minerals from the vegetables.
- It's low in fat, making it gentle on the gallbladder, and the fiber from the veggies promotes healthy digestion.

Preparation Time: Approximately 10 minutes

2: Greek Yogurt Parfait

Ingredients:

- 1/2 cup plain Greek yogurt
- 1/4 cup fresh berries (such as strawberries, blueberries, or raspberries)

- 2 tablespoons granola
- 1 teaspoon honey (optional)

Instructions:

- In a serving glass or bowl, layer half of the Greek yogurt.
- Add half of the berries on top of the yogurt layer.
- Sprinkle half of the granola over the berries.
- Repeat the layers with the remaining yogurt, berries, and granola.
- Drizzle honey over the top if desired.
- Serve immediately.

Health Benefits:

- This Greek yogurt parfait is rich in protein from the Greek yogurt and contains antioxidants and fiber from the berries.
- The granola adds a crunchy texture and provides additional fiber and energy.

Preparation Time: Approximately 5 minutes

3: Banana Oatmeal

Ingredients:

- 1/2 cup rolled oats
- 1 cup water or milk (almond milk or skim milk)
- 1 ripe banana, mashed
- 1 tablespoon honey (optional)
- 1/2 teaspoon cinnamon (optional)
- Chopped nuts or seeds for topping (optional)

Instructions:

- In a small saucepan, bring the water or milk to a boil.
- Stir in the rolled oats and reduce the heat to low.
- Simmer for 5-7 minutes, stirring occasionally, until the oats are cooked and the mixture has thickened.
- Remove from heat and stir in the mashed banana, honey (if using), and cinnamon (if using).
- Transfer the oatmeal to a bowl and top with chopped nuts or seeds if desired.
- Serve warm.

Health Benefits:

- This banana oatmeal is a hearty and nutritious breakfast option.
- Oats are high in fiber, which aids digestion and promotes gallbladder health.
- Bananas provide natural sweetness and potassium, while cinnamon adds flavor without extra calories.

Preparation Time: Approximately 10 minutes

4: Avocado Toast

Ingredients:

- 1 slice whole-grain bread
- 1/2 ripe avocado
- 1 teaspoon lemon juice
- Salt and pepper to taste
- Red pepper flakes (optional)
- Chopped fresh herbs (such as cilantro or parsley) for garnish (optional)

Instructions:

- Toast the slice of whole-grain bread until golden brown.
- In a small bowl, mash the ripe avocado with lemon juice, salt, and pepper until smooth.
- Spread the mashed avocado evenly onto the toasted bread.
- Sprinkle with red pepper flakes for a hint of spice if desired.
- Garnish with chopped fresh herbs for added flavor and presentation.
- Serve immediately.

Health Benefits:

- Avocado toast is a nutrient-rich breakfast option. Avocados are high in healthy fats, which are beneficial for gallbladder health.
- Whole-grain bread provides fiber, and lemon juice adds a refreshing flavor while aiding digestion.

Preparation Time: Approximately 5 minutes

5: Spinach and Feta Egg Muffins

Ingredients:

- 4 eggs
- 1 cup fresh spinach, chopped
- 1/4 cup crumbled feta cheese
- Salt and pepper to taste
- Cooking spray or olive oil for greasing muffin tin

Instructions:

- Preheat your oven to 350°F (175°C). Grease a muffin tin with cooking spray or olive oil.
- In a mixing bowl, whisk together the eggs until well beaten.
- Stir in the chopped spinach and crumbled feta cheese. Season with salt and pepper to taste.
- Pour the egg mixture evenly into the prepared muffin tin, filling each cup about 3/4 full.
- Bake in the preheated oven for 20-25 minutes, or until the egg muffins are set and lightly golden on top.

- Allow the egg muffins to cool for a few minutes before removing them from the muffin tin. Serve warm.

Health Benefits:

- These spinach and feta egg muffins are packed with protein from the eggs and calcium from the feta cheese.
- Spinach adds fiber and essential nutrients like vitamins A and C, while being gentle on the gallbladder.

Preparation Time: Approximately 30 minutes

6: Chia Seed Pudding

Ingredients:

- 1/4 cup chia seeds
- 1 cup unsweetened almond milk or coconut milk
- 1 tablespoon honey or maple syrup (optional)
- 1/2 teaspoon vanilla extract
- Fresh fruit for topping (such as berries or sliced banana)

Instructions:

- In a mixing bowl or jar, combine the chia seeds, almond milk or coconut milk, honey or maple syrup (if using), and vanilla extract. Stir well to combine.
- Cover the bowl or jar and refrigerate for at least 2 hours or overnight, allowing the chia seeds to absorb the liquid and thicken.
- Once the chia pudding has set, give it a good stir to break up any clumps.
- Spoon the chia pudding into serving bowls and top with fresh fruit of your choice.
- Serve chilled.

Health Benefits:

- Chia seed pudding is a nutritious and satisfying breakfast option.
- Chia seeds are rich in fiber, omega-3 fatty acids, and antioxidants, which support digestive health and reduce inflammation.
- Almond milk or coconut milk provide creamy texture without excess fat.

Preparation Time: Approximately 2 hours (includes chilling time)

7: Cottage Cheese Pancakes

Ingredients:

- 1/2 cup cottage cheese
- 2 eggs
- 1/4 cup oat flour (you can make your own by blending rolled oats)
- 1/2 teaspoon baking powder
- 1/2 teaspoon vanilla extract
- Cooking spray or butter for greasing the pan

Instructions:

- In a blender or food processor, combine the cottage cheese, eggs, oat flour, baking powder, and vanilla extract. Blend until smooth.
- Heat a non-stick skillet or griddle over medium heat and lightly grease with cooking spray or butter.
- Pour the pancake batter onto the skillet to form small pancakes (about 2-3 tablespoons of batter per pancake).

- Cook for 2-3 minutes, or until bubbles form on the surface of the pancakes and the edges begin to set.
- Flip the pancakes and cook for an additional 1-2 minutes, or until golden brown on both sides.
- Repeat with the remaining batter, greasing the skillet as needed.
- Serve the pancakes warm with your choice of toppings, such as fresh fruit, Greek yogurt, or a drizzle of honey.

Health Benefits:

- Cottage cheese pancakes are a protein-rich breakfast option that is gentle on the gallbladder.
- Cottage cheese provides high-quality protein, while oat flour adds fiber and complex carbohydrates.
- These pancakes are also lower in fat compared to traditional pancakes made with butter or oil.

Preparation Time: Approximately 15 minutes

8: Quinoa Breakfast Bowl

Ingredients:

- 1/2 cup cooked quinoa

- 1/4 cup unsweetened almond milk or coconut milk
- 1 tablespoon almond butter or peanut butter
- 1/2 teaspoon honey or maple syrup (optional)
- Fresh fruit for topping (such as sliced banana, berries, or diced apple)
- Chopped nuts or seeds for topping (such as almonds, walnuts, or pumpkin seeds)
- Cinnamon or nutmeg for flavor (optional)

Instructions:

- In a saucepan, combine the cooked quinoa and almond milk or coconut milk over medium heat. Stir in the almond butter or peanut butter and honey or maple syrup (if using).
- Cook for 2-3 minutes, or until the quinoa is heated through and the mixture is creamy.
- Transfer the quinoa mixture to a serving bowl.
- Top with fresh fruit, chopped nuts or seeds, and a sprinkle of cinnamon or nutmeg if desired.
- Serve warm.

Health Benefits:

- Quinoa breakfast bowls are a nutritious and filling option for a gallbladder-friendly breakfast.
- Quinoa is a complete protein, meaning it contains all nine essential amino acids. It's also high in fiber, vitamins, and minerals, making it a great choice for digestive health and overall well-being.

Preparation Time: Approximately 10 minutes

9: Apple Cinnamon Overnight Oats

Ingredients:

- 1/2 cup rolled oats
- 1/2 cup unsweetened almond milk or any milk of your choice
- 1/2 cup diced apple (about half a medium-sized apple)
- 1 tablespoon maple syrup or honey (optional)
- 1/2 teaspoon ground cinnamon
- 1 tablespoon chopped nuts (such as walnuts or almonds) for topping (optional)

Instructions:

- In a jar or bowl, combine the rolled oats, almond milk, diced apple, maple syrup or honey (if using), and ground cinnamon. Stir well to mix all ingredients.
- Cover the jar or bowl and refrigerate overnight, or for at least 4 hours, to allow the oats to soften and absorb the liquid.
- Before serving, give the overnight oats a good stir. If desired, add a splash of almond milk to adjust the consistency.
- Top with chopped nuts for extra crunch and flavor.
- Serve chilled.

Health Benefits:

- This apple cinnamon overnight oats recipe is rich in fiber from the oats and apple, which helps promote digestive health and may reduce the risk of gallbladder issues.
- The combination of complex carbohydrates and protein from the oats and almond milk provides sustained energy throughout the morning.

Preparation Time: Approximately 5 minutes (plus chilling time)

10: Sweet Potato Breakfast Hash

Ingredients:

- 1 medium sweet potato, peeled and diced
- 1/2 small onion, diced
- 1/2 bell pepper, diced
- 1 tablespoon olive oil or coconut oil
- Salt and pepper to taste
- 2 eggs
- Fresh herbs for garnish (such as parsley or cilantro)

Instructions:

- Heat olive oil or coconut oil in a skillet over medium heat.
- Add the diced sweet potato to the skillet and cook for about 5 minutes, stirring occasionally, until slightly softened.
- Add the diced onion and bell pepper to the skillet and continue cooking for another 5-7 minutes, or until the vegetables are tender and lightly caramelized.

- Season with salt and pepper to taste.
- Create two small wells in the hash mixture and crack an egg into each well.
- Cover the skillet and cook for 3-5 minutes, or until the eggs are cooked to your desired doneness.
- Garnish with fresh herbs before serving.
- Serve hot.

Health Benefits:

- This sweet potato breakfast hash is packed with vitamins, minerals, and fiber from the sweet potatoes, onion, and bell pepper.
- Eggs provide high-quality protein, while olive oil or coconut oil adds healthy fats.
- This hearty breakfast option is both satisfying and nutritious, making it an excellent choice for gallbladder health.

Preparation Time: Approximately 20 minutes

Gallbladder Diet Lunch Recipes for Beginners

1: Grilled Lemon Herb Chicken Salad

Ingredients:

- 2 boneless, skinless chicken breasts
- 2 tablespoons olive oil
- 1 lemon, juiced and zested
- 2 cloves garlic, minced
- 1 teaspoon dried thyme
- 1 teaspoon dried oregano
- Salt and pepper to taste
- 4 cups mixed salad greens
- 1/2 cucumber, sliced
- 1/2 cup cherry tomatoes, halved
- 1/4 cup sliced red onion
- 2 tablespoons balsamic vinaigrette dressing

Instructions:

- In a small bowl, whisk together olive oil, lemon juice and zest, minced garlic, dried thyme, dried oregano, salt, and pepper to make the marinade.

- Place chicken breasts in a shallow dish and pour the marinade over them. Allow to marinate for at least 30 minutes in the refrigerator.
- Preheat grill to medium-high heat. Grill the chicken breasts for 6-8 minutes on each side, or until cooked through and no longer pink in the center. Remove from heat and let rest for a few minutes before slicing.
- Meanwhile, arrange mixed salad greens on serving plates and top with sliced cucumber, cherry tomatoes, and red onion.
- Slice grilled chicken breasts and place on top of the salad.
- Drizzle with balsamic vinaigrette dressing.
- Serve immediately.

Health Benefits:

- This grilled lemon herb chicken salad is rich in lean protein from the chicken breasts and packed with vitamins, minerals, and antioxidants from the mixed salad greens and vegetables.

- Olive oil provides healthy fats, while lemon adds a refreshing flavor.

Preparation Time: Approximately 40 minutes (including marinating time)

2: Quinoa and Black Bean Stuffed Bell Peppers

Ingredients:

- 4 large bell peppers (any color)
- 1 cup cooked quinoa
- 1 cup canned black beans, drained and rinsed
- 1 cup diced tomatoes
- 1/2 cup diced red onion
- 1/2 cup corn kernels (fresh, canned, or frozen)
- 1/2 teaspoon ground cumin
- 1/2 teaspoon chili powder
- Salt and pepper to taste
- 1/2 cup shredded cheddar cheese (optional)
- Fresh cilantro for garnish (optional)

Instructions:

- Preheat oven to 375°F (190°C). Slice the tops off the bell peppers and remove the seeds and membranes from the inside.
- In a large mixing bowl, combine cooked quinoa, black beans, diced tomatoes, diced red onion, corn kernels, ground cumin, chili powder, salt, and pepper. Mix well to combine.
- Stuff each bell pepper with the quinoa and black bean mixture, pressing down gently to pack the filling.
- Place stuffed bell peppers in a baking dish and cover with foil.
- Bake in the preheated oven for 25-30 minutes, or until the peppers are tender.
- If using shredded cheese, remove the foil from the baking dish and sprinkle cheese over the tops of the stuffed peppers. Return to the oven and bake for an additional 5 minutes, or until the cheese is melted and bubbly.
- Garnish with fresh cilantro before serving, if desired.
- Serve hot.

Health Benefits:

- These quinoa and black bean stuffed bell peppers are a nutritious and satisfying lunch option.
- Quinoa provides protein and fiber, while black beans add additional protein and essential nutrients.
- Bell peppers are rich in vitamins and antioxidants, making this dish a powerhouse of nutrition.

Preparation Time: Approximately 45 minutes

3: Baked Salmon with Roasted Vegetables

Ingredients:

- 2 salmon fillets
- 2 tablespoons olive oil
- 1 lemon, juiced
- 2 cloves garlic, minced
- 1 teaspoon dried dill
- Salt and pepper to taste
- 2 cups mixed vegetables (such as carrots, broccoli, and cauliflower), chopped
- Cooking spray
- Fresh parsley for garnish (optional)

Instructions:

- Preheat oven to 400°F (200°C). Line a baking sheet with parchment paper and lightly coat with cooking spray.
- In a small bowl, whisk together olive oil, lemon juice, minced garlic, dried dill, salt, and pepper to make the marinade.
- Place salmon fillets on the prepared baking sheet. Brush the marinade over the salmon.
- In a separate bowl, toss mixed vegetables with a tablespoon of olive oil and season with salt and pepper.
- Spread the mixed vegetables around the salmon on the baking sheet.
- Bake in the preheated oven for 15-20 minutes, or until the salmon is cooked through and flakes easily with a fork, and the vegetables are tender and lightly browned.
- Garnish with fresh parsley before serving, if desired.
- Serve hot.

Health Benefits:

- This baked salmon with roasted vegetables dish is rich in omega-3 fatty acids from the salmon, which are beneficial for gallbladder health.
- The mixed vegetables provide fiber, vitamins, and minerals, while the olive oil adds healthy fats and flavor.

Preparation Time: Approximately 25 minutes

4: Lentil and Vegetable Soup

Ingredients:

- 1 cup dried green or brown lentils, rinsed and drained
- 4 cups vegetable broth
- 1 onion, chopped
- 2 carrots, diced
- 2 celery stalks, diced
- 2 cloves garlic, minced
- 1 teaspoon dried thyme
- 1 teaspoon dried rosemary
- Salt and pepper to taste
- 2 cups chopped spinach or kale

- 1 tablespoon lemon juice
- Fresh parsley for garnish (optional)

Instructions:

- In a large pot, combine lentils, vegetable broth, chopped onion, diced carrots, diced celery, minced garlic, dried thyme, and dried rosemary. Season with salt and pepper to taste.
- Bring the soup to a boil over medium-high heat. Reduce heat to low, cover, and simmer for 25-30 minutes, or until the lentils and vegetables are tender.
- Stir in chopped spinach or kale and simmer for an additional 5 minutes, or until wilted.
- Remove the soup from heat and stir in lemon juice.
- Ladle the soup into serving bowls and garnish with fresh parsley before serving, if desired.
- Serve hot.

Health Benefits:

- This lentil and vegetable soup is a nutritious and comforting lunch option.

- Lentils are rich in fiber and protein, which promote digestive health and help maintain stable blood sugar levels.
- The vegetables add vitamins, minerals, and antioxidants, while the lemon juice provides a refreshing flavor boost.

Preparation Time: Approximately 40 minutes

5: Turkey and Avocado Wrap

Ingredients:

- 2 large whole-grain tortillas or wraps
- 1/2 lb sliced turkey breast
- 1 ripe avocado, sliced
- 1 cup mixed salad greens
- 1/2 cup shredded carrots
- 1/4 cup sliced cucumber
- 2 tablespoons hummus or Greek yogurt spread
- Salt and pepper to taste

Instructions:

- Lay out the tortillas or wraps on a clean surface.

- Spread a tablespoon of hummus or Greek yogurt spread evenly over each tortilla.
- Layer sliced turkey breast, avocado slices, mixed salad greens, shredded carrots, and sliced cucumber on top of the spread.
- Season with salt and pepper to taste.
- Roll up the tortillas tightly, tucking in the sides as you go.
- Slice each wrap in half diagonally and serve.

Health Benefits:

- This turkey and avocado wrap is a balanced and satisfying lunch option.
- Turkey provides lean protein, while avocado offers healthy fats and fiber.
- Whole-grain tortillas add complex carbohydrates and additional fiber, making this meal gentle on the gallbladder and nutritious.

Preparation Time: Approximately 10 minutes

6: Quinoa Salad with Lemon Herb Dressing

Ingredients:

- 1 cup cooked quinoa, cooled
- 1 cup chopped cucumber
- 1 cup halved cherry tomatoes
- 1/2 cup diced red bell pepper
- 1/4 cup chopped fresh parsley
- 1/4 cup chopped fresh mint
- 1/4 cup crumbled feta cheese (optional)
- 2 tablespoons extra-virgin olive oil
- 1 lemon, juiced and zested
- 1 clove garlic, minced
- Salt and pepper to taste

Instructions:

- In a large mixing bowl, combine cooked quinoa, chopped cucumber, cherry tomatoes, diced red bell pepper, chopped fresh parsley, chopped fresh mint, and crumbled feta cheese (if using).
- In a small bowl, whisk together extra-virgin olive oil, lemon juice and zest, minced garlic, salt, and pepper to make the dressing.

- Pour the dressing over the quinoa salad and toss gently to coat.
- Taste and adjust seasoning as needed.
- Serve immediately or refrigerate for later.

Health Benefits:

- This quinoa salad with lemon herb dressing is packed with fiber, protein, vitamins, and antioxidants.
- Quinoa provides a complete source of protein, while vegetables add essential nutrients and fiber.
- The lemon herb dressing adds bright flavor without excess fat, making this salad both delicious and gallbladder-friendly.

Preparation Time: Approximately 20 minutes (not including quinoa cooking time)

7: Chickpea Salad Sandwich

Ingredients:

- 1 can (15 ounces) chickpeas (garbanzo beans), drained and rinsed
- 1/4 cup diced red onion
- 1/4 cup diced celery

- 1/4 cup diced bell pepper (any color)
- 2 tablespoons chopped fresh parsley
- 2 tablespoons Greek yogurt or hummus
- 1 tablespoon lemon juice
- 1 teaspoon Dijon mustard
- Salt and pepper to taste
- Lettuce leaves
- Whole-grain bread or sandwich wraps

Instructions:

- In a mixing bowl, mash the chickpeas with a fork or potato masher until coarse.
- Add diced red onion, celery, bell pepper, chopped parsley, Greek yogurt or hummus, lemon juice, Dijon mustard, salt, and pepper to the mashed chickpeas. Mix until well combined.
- Taste and adjust seasoning as needed.
- To assemble the sandwiches, spread a generous portion of the chickpea salad onto whole-grain bread slices or wraps.
- Top with lettuce leaves and another slice of bread or fold the wrap.

- Slice the sandwiches in half and serve.

Health Benefits:

- This chickpea salad sandwich is a plant-based alternative to traditional tuna or chicken salad sandwiches.
- Chickpeas provide protein and fiber, while vegetables add vitamins, minerals, and antioxidants.
- Greek yogurt or hummus adds creaminess without excess fat, making this sandwich both nutritious and gallbladder-friendly.

Preparation Time: Approximately 15 minutes

8: Zucchini Noodles with Pesto and Cherry Tomatoes

Ingredients:

- 2 medium zucchini, spiralized into noodles
- 1 cup cherry tomatoes, halved
- 2 tablespoons pesto sauce (store-bought or homemade)
- 1 tablespoon olive oil
- 2 cloves garlic, minced

- Salt and pepper to taste
- Grated Parmesan cheese for garnish (optional)
- Fresh basil leaves for garnish (optional)

Instructions:

- Heat olive oil in a large skillet over medium heat. Add minced garlic and cook for 1-2 minutes, or until fragrant.
- Add spiralized zucchini noodles to the skillet and sauté for 2-3 minutes, or until just tender.
- Stir in halved cherry tomatoes and cook for another 1-2 minutes, or until heated through.
- Remove the skillet from heat and stir in pesto sauce until the noodles and tomatoes are evenly coated.
- Taste and adjust seasoning with salt and pepper as needed.
- Transfer the zucchini noodles with pesto and cherry tomatoes to serving plates.
- Garnish with grated Parmesan cheese and fresh basil leaves, if desired.
- Serve immediately.

Health Benefits:

- This zucchini noodles with pesto and cherry tomatoes dish is a light and flavorful lunch option.
- Zucchini noodles provide a low-carb, low-calorie alternative to traditional pasta, while cherry tomatoes add vitamins, minerals, and antioxidants.
- Pesto sauce adds rich flavor without excess fat, making this meal both delicious and gallbladder-friendly.

Preparation Time: Approximately 15 minutes

9: Tuna Salad Lettuce Wraps

Ingredients:

- 1 can (5 ounces) tuna, drained
- 2 tablespoons Greek yogurt or mayonnaise
- 1 tablespoon lemon juice
- 1/4 cup diced celery
- 1/4 cup diced red onion
- Salt and pepper to taste
- Lettuce leaves (such as butter lettuce or romaine hearts)

- Sliced cucumber and avocado for topping (optional)

Instructions:

- In a mixing bowl, combine drained tuna, Greek yogurt or mayonnaise, lemon juice, diced celery, and diced red onion. Mix until well combined.
- Season the tuna salad with salt and pepper to taste. Adjust seasoning as needed.
- Place a spoonful of tuna salad onto each lettuce leaf.
- Add sliced cucumber and avocado on top of the tuna salad, if desired.
- Roll up the lettuce leaves to form wraps.
- Serve immediately.

Health Benefits:

- These tuna salad lettuce wraps are a light and protein-packed lunch option.
- Tuna provides lean protein, while Greek yogurt or mayonnaise adds creaminess without excess fat.
- Lettuce leaves serve as a low-carb alternative to traditional wraps or bread, making this meal gentle on the gallbladder and nutritious.

Preparation Time: Approximately 10 minutes

10: Veggie Stir-Fry with Brown Rice

Ingredients:

- 1 cup cooked brown rice
- 2 cups mixed vegetables (such as bell peppers, broccoli, carrots, snap peas, and mushrooms), sliced or diced
- 2 tablespoons low-sodium soy sauce or tamari
- 1 tablespoon olive oil
- 2 cloves garlic, minced
- 1 teaspoon grated fresh ginger
- 1 tablespoon rice vinegar
- 1 teaspoon sesame oil (optional)
- Sesame seeds and chopped green onions for garnish (optional)

Instructions:

- Heat olive oil in a large skillet or wok over medium-high heat.
- Add minced garlic and grated ginger to the skillet and cook for 1 minute, or until fragrant.

- Add mixed vegetables to the skillet and stir-fry for 4-5 minutes, or until tender-crisp.
- In a small bowl, whisk together low-sodium soy sauce or tamari, rice vinegar, and sesame oil (if using).
- Pour the sauce over the vegetables in the skillet and toss to coat evenly.
- Add cooked brown rice to the skillet and stir-fry for another 2-3 minutes, or until heated through.
- Remove the skillet from heat and transfer the veggie stir-fry with brown rice to serving plates.
- Garnish with sesame seeds and chopped green onions, if desired.
- Serve hot.

Health Benefits:

- This veggie stir-fry with brown rice is a nutritious and filling lunch option.
- Brown rice provides complex carbohydrates and fiber, while mixed vegetables add vitamins, minerals, and antioxidants.

- The stir-fry is seasoned with a flavorful sauce made with low-sodium soy sauce, garlic, ginger, and rice vinegar, making it both delicious and gallbladder-friendly.

Preparation Time: Approximately 20 minutes

Gallbladder Diet Dinner Recipes for Beginners

1: Baked Lemon Herb Salmon

Ingredients:

- 2 salmon fillets
- 2 tablespoons olive oil
- 1 lemon, juiced and zested
- 2 cloves garlic, minced
- 1 teaspoon dried thyme
- 1 teaspoon dried rosemary
- Salt and pepper to taste
- Sliced lemon for garnish (optional)
- Fresh parsley for garnish (optional)

Instructions:

- Preheat oven to 375°F (190°C). Line a baking sheet with parchment paper.
- In a small bowl, whisk together olive oil, lemon juice and zest, minced garlic, dried thyme, dried rosemary, salt, and pepper to make the marinade.
- Place salmon fillets on the prepared baking sheet. Brush the marinade over the salmon.
- Bake in the preheated oven for 12-15 minutes, or until the salmon is cooked through and flakes easily with a fork.
- Garnish with sliced lemon and fresh parsley before serving, if desired.
- Serve hot.

Health Benefits:

- This baked lemon herb salmon is rich in omega-3 fatty acids, which are beneficial for gallbladder health.
- Salmon is also a good source of lean protein and essential nutrients.

- The herbs and lemon add flavor without extra calories or fat, making this dish both delicious and gallbladder-friendly.

Preparation Time: Approximately 20 minutes

2: Quinoa and Vegetable Stir-Fry

Ingredients:

- 1 cup uncooked quinoa
- 2 cups water or vegetable broth
- 2 tablespoons olive oil
- 2 cloves garlic, minced
- 1 onion, diced
- 2 carrots, sliced
- 1 bell pepper, sliced
- 1 cup broccoli florets
- 1 cup snap peas
- 2 tablespoons low-sodium soy sauce or tamari
- 1 tablespoon rice vinegar
- Salt and pepper to taste
- Sesame seeds for garnish (optional)
- Chopped green onions for garnish (optional)

Instructions:

- Rinse quinoa under cold water. In a medium saucepan, bring water or vegetable broth to a boil. Add quinoa, reduce heat to low, cover, and simmer for 15-20 minutes, or until quinoa is cooked and water is absorbed. Remove from heat and let it sit, covered, for 5 minutes. Fluff with a fork.
- In a large skillet or wok, heat olive oil over medium-high heat. Add minced garlic and diced onion, and cook for 1-2 minutes, or until fragrant.
- Add sliced carrots, bell pepper, broccoli florets, and snap peas to the skillet. Stir-fry for 4-5 minutes, or until vegetables are tender-crisp.
- In a small bowl, whisk together low-sodium soy sauce or tamari, and rice vinegar. Pour the sauce over the vegetables in the skillet and toss to coat evenly.
- Add cooked quinoa to the skillet and stir-fry for another 2-3 minutes, or until heated through.
- Season with salt and pepper to taste.
- Garnish with sesame seeds and chopped green onions before serving, if desired.
- Serve hot.

Health Benefits:

- This quinoa and vegetable stir-fry is a nutritious and satisfying dinner option.
- Quinoa provides protein, fiber, and complex carbohydrates, while vegetables add vitamins, minerals, and antioxidants.
- The stir-fry is seasoned with a flavorful sauce made with low-sodium soy sauce or tamari, and rice vinegar, making it both delicious and gallbladder-friendly.

Preparation Time: Approximately 30 minutes

3: Roasted Chicken with Sweet Potatoes and Broccoli

Ingredients:

- 2 boneless, skinless chicken breasts
- 2 medium sweet potatoes, peeled and diced
- 2 cups broccoli florets
- 2 tablespoons olive oil
- 2 cloves garlic, minced
- 1 teaspoon dried thyme

- Salt and pepper to taste
- Fresh lemon wedges for serving (optional)

Instructions:

- Preheat oven to 400°F (200°C). Line a baking sheet with parchment paper.
- In a small bowl, mix together olive oil, minced garlic, dried thyme, salt, and pepper.
- Place chicken breasts on one side of the prepared baking sheet. Brush both sides of the chicken with the olive oil mixture.
- Place diced sweet potatoes and broccoli florets on the other side of the baking sheet. Drizzle with remaining olive oil mixture and toss to coat.
- Roast in the preheated oven for 25-30 minutes, or until chicken is cooked through and vegetables are tender, flipping the chicken halfway through cooking.
- Remove from oven and let the chicken rest for a few minutes before slicing.

- Serve the roasted chicken with sweet potatoes and broccoli alongside fresh lemon wedges for squeezing over the chicken, if desired.
- Serve hot.

Health Benefits:

- This roasted chicken with sweet potatoes and broccoli is a well-balanced dinner option.
- Chicken provides lean protein, while sweet potatoes and broccoli offer vitamins, minerals, and fiber.
- Olive oil adds healthy fats, while garlic and thyme add flavor without excess calories or fat.

Preparation Time: Approximately 40 minutes

4: Lentil and Vegetable Soup

Ingredients:

- 1 cup dried green or brown lentils, rinsed and drained
- 4 cups vegetable broth
- 1 onion, chopped
- 2 carrots, diced
- 2 celery stalks, diced
- 2 cloves garlic, minced

- 1 teaspoon dried thyme
- 1 teaspoon dried rosemary
- Salt and pepper to taste
- 2 cups chopped spinach or kale
- 1 tablespoon lemon juice
- Fresh parsley for garnish (optional)

Instructions:

- In a large pot, combine lentils, vegetable broth, chopped onion, diced carrots, diced celery, minced garlic, dried thyme, and dried rosemary. Season with salt and pepper to taste.
- Bring the soup to a boil over medium-high heat. Reduce heat to low, cover, and simmer for 25-30 minutes, or until the lentils and vegetables are tender.
- Stir in chopped spinach or kale and simmer for an additional 5 minutes, or until wilted.
- Remove the soup from heat and stir in lemon juice.
- Ladle the soup into serving bowls and garnish with fresh parsley before serving, if desired.
- Serve hot.

Health Benefits:

- This lentil and vegetable soup is a nutritious and comforting dinner option.
- Lentils provide protein and fiber, while vegetables add vitamins, minerals, and antioxidants.
- The soup is seasoned with herbs and lemon juice, making it flavorful without excess calories or fat.

Preparation Time: Approximately 40 minutes

5: Turkey and Vegetable Skillet

Ingredients:

- 1 lb ground turkey
- 1 tablespoon olive oil
- 1 onion, diced
- 2 cloves garlic, minced
- 2 carrots, diced
- 1 bell pepper, diced
- 1 zucchini, diced
- 1 cup cherry tomatoes, halved
- 1 teaspoon dried oregano
- 1 teaspoon dried basil

- Salt and pepper to taste
- Cooked brown rice or quinoa for serving (optional)

Instructions:

- Heat olive oil in a large skillet over medium heat. Add diced onion and minced garlic, and sauté until fragrant, about 1-2 minutes.
- Add ground turkey to the skillet and cook until browned, breaking it up with a spoon as it cooks.
- Add diced carrots, bell pepper, and zucchini to the skillet. Cook for 5-7 minutes, or until vegetables are tender.
- Stir in halved cherry tomatoes, dried oregano, dried basil, salt, and pepper. Cook for an additional 2-3 minutes, until tomatoes are slightly softened.
- Taste and adjust seasoning as needed.
- Serve the turkey and vegetable skillet on its own or over cooked brown rice or quinoa for a complete meal.

Health Benefits:

- This turkey and vegetable skillet is a nutritious and easy-to-make dinner option.

- Turkey provides lean protein, while vegetables add vitamins, minerals, and fiber. This dish is low in fat and gentle on the gallbladder, making it a great choice for a healthy dinner.

Preparation Time: Approximately 30 minutes

6: Stuffed Bell Peppers with Quinoa and Black Beans

Ingredients:

- 4 large bell peppers (any color)
- 1 cup cooked quinoa
- 1 cup canned black beans, drained and rinsed
- 1 cup diced tomatoes
- 1/2 cup diced red onion
- 1/2 cup corn kernels (fresh, canned, or frozen)
- 1 teaspoon ground cumin
- 1 teaspoon chili powder
- Salt and pepper to taste
- 1/2 cup shredded cheddar cheese (optional)
- Fresh cilantro for garnish (optional)

Instructions:

- Preheat oven to 375°F (190°C). Slice the tops off the bell peppers and remove the seeds and membranes from the inside.
- In a large mixing bowl, combine cooked quinoa, black beans, diced tomatoes, diced red onion, corn kernels, ground cumin, chili powder, salt, and pepper. Mix well to combine.
- Stuff each bell pepper with the quinoa and black bean mixture, pressing down gently to pack the filling.
- Place stuffed bell peppers in a baking dish and cover with foil.
- Bake in the preheated oven for 25-30 minutes, or until the peppers are tender.
- If using shredded cheese, remove the foil from the baking dish and sprinkle cheese over the tops of the stuffed peppers. Return to the oven and bake for an additional 5 minutes, or until the cheese is melted and bubbly.
- Garnish with fresh cilantro before serving, if desired.
- Serve hot.

Health Benefits:

- These stuffed bell peppers with quinoa and black beans are a nutritious and satisfying dinner option.
- Bell peppers provide vitamins and antioxidants, while quinoa and black beans offer protein, fiber, and essential nutrients.
- This dish is low in fat and gentle on the gallbladder, making it a great choice for a healthy dinner.

Preparation Time: Approximately 45 minutes

7: Grilled Lemon Herb Chicken with Steamed Vegetables

Ingredients:

- 2 boneless, skinless chicken breasts
- 2 tablespoons olive oil
- 1 lemon, juiced and zested
- 2 cloves garlic, minced
- 1 teaspoon dried thyme
- 1 teaspoon dried rosemary
- Salt and pepper to taste

- Assorted vegetables for steaming (such as broccoli, carrots, and cauliflower)
- Fresh parsley for garnish (optional)

Instructions:

- In a small bowl, whisk together olive oil, lemon juice and zest, minced garlic, dried thyme, dried rosemary, salt, and pepper to make the marinade.
- Place chicken breasts in a shallow dish and pour the marinade over them. Allow to marinate for at least 30 minutes in the refrigerator.
- Preheat grill to medium-high heat. Grill the chicken breasts for 6-8 minutes on each side, or until cooked through and no longer pink in the center. Remove from heat and let rest for a few minutes before slicing.
- While the chicken is grilling, prepare the steamed vegetables by placing them in a steamer basket over boiling water. Steam for 5-7 minutes, or until tender-crisp.
- Arrange the sliced grilled chicken and steamed vegetables on serving plates.

- Garnish with fresh parsley before serving, if desired.
- Serve hot.

Health Benefits:

- This grilled lemon herb chicken with steamed vegetables is a healthy and balanced dinner option.
- Chicken provides lean protein, while vegetables offer vitamins, minerals, and fiber.
- The marinade adds flavor without excess calories or fat, making this dish both delicious and gallbladder-friendly.

Preparation Time: Approximately 40 minutes

8: Baked Cod with Roasted Asparagus

Ingredients:

- 2 cod fillets
- 2 tablespoons olive oil
- 1 lemon, juiced and zested
- 2 cloves garlic, minced
- Salt and pepper to taste
- 1 bunch asparagus, woody ends trimmed
- Lemon wedges for serving (optional)

Instructions:

- Preheat oven to 400°F (200°C). Line a baking sheet with parchment paper.
- In a small bowl, whisk together olive oil, lemon juice and zest, minced garlic, salt, and pepper.
- Place cod fillets on the prepared baking sheet. Brush both sides of the cod with the olive oil mixture.
- Arrange asparagus spears on the baking sheet around the cod fillets. Drizzle with any remaining olive oil mixture.
- Bake in the preheated oven for 12-15 minutes, or until the cod is opaque and flakes easily with a fork, and the asparagus is tender.
- Remove from oven and let the cod and asparagus rest for a few minutes before serving.
- Serve hot with lemon wedges on the side, if desired.

Health Benefits:

- This baked cod with roasted asparagus is a light and nutritious dinner option.

- Cod is a lean source of protein and omega-3 fatty acids, while asparagus offers vitamins, minerals, and fiber.
- The lemon and garlic-infused olive oil adds flavor without excess calories or fat, making this dish both delicious and gallbladder-friendly.

Preparation Time: Approximately 20 minutes

9: Vegetarian Lentil Soup

Ingredients:

- 1 cup dried green or brown lentils, rinsed and drained
- 4 cups vegetable broth
- 1 onion, chopped
- 2 carrots, diced
- 2 celery stalks, diced
- 2 cloves garlic, minced
- 1 teaspoon dried thyme
- 1 teaspoon dried rosemary
- Salt and pepper to taste
- 2 cups chopped spinach or kale
- 1 tablespoon lemon juice

- Fresh parsley for garnish (optional)

Instructions:

- In a large pot, combine lentils, vegetable broth, chopped onion, diced carrots, diced celery, minced garlic, dried thyme, and dried rosemary. Season with salt and pepper to taste.
- Bring the soup to a boil over medium-high heat. Reduce heat to low, cover, and simmer for 25-30 minutes, or until the lentils and vegetables are tender.
- Stir in chopped spinach or kale and simmer for an additional 5 minutes, or until wilted.
- Remove the soup from heat and stir in lemon juice.
- Ladle the soup into serving bowls and garnish with fresh parsley before serving, if desired.
- Serve hot.

Health Benefits:

- This vegetarian lentil soup is hearty and packed with nutrients.
- Lentils provide protein and fiber, while vegetables add vitamins, minerals, and antioxidants.

- The soup is seasoned with herbs and lemon juice, making it flavorful without excess calories or fat. This dish is gentle on the gallbladder and suitable for vegetarians.

Preparation Time: Approximately 40 minutes

10: Baked Chicken and Vegetable Sheet Pan Dinner

Ingredients:

- 2 boneless, skinless chicken breasts
- 2 tablespoons olive oil
- 2 cloves garlic, minced
- 1 teaspoon dried oregano
- 1 teaspoon dried thyme
- Salt and pepper to taste
- 1 cup baby potatoes, halved
- 1 cup baby carrots
- 1 cup Brussels sprouts, halved
- 1 bell pepper, sliced
- Fresh parsley for garnish (optional)

Instructions:

- Preheat oven to 400°F (200°C). Line a baking sheet with parchment paper.
- In a small bowl, whisk together olive oil, minced garlic, dried oregano, dried thyme, salt, and pepper.
- Place chicken breasts on the prepared baking sheet. Brush both sides of the chicken with the olive oil mixture.
- In a large mixing bowl, toss halved baby potatoes, baby carrots, Brussels sprouts, and sliced bell pepper with the remaining olive oil mixture until evenly coated.
- Arrange the vegetables around the chicken on the baking sheet.
- Bake in the preheated oven for 25-30 minutes, or until the chicken is cooked through and vegetables are tender and lightly browned.
- Remove from oven and let the chicken and vegetables rest for a few minutes before serving.
- Garnish with fresh parsley before serving, if desired.
- Serve hot.

Health Benefits:

- This baked chicken and vegetable sheet pan dinner is a simple and wholesome meal.
- Chicken provides lean protein, while vegetables offer vitamins, minerals, and fiber.
- Baking the ingredients together makes for easy cleanup and ensures all components are cooked perfectly. This dish is gentle on the gallbladder and suitable for a balanced dinner.

Preparation Time: Approximately 40 minutes

Gallbladder Diet Snacks Recipes for Beginners

1: Greek Yogurt Parfait with Berries

Ingredients:

- 1 cup plain Greek yogurt
- 1/2 cup mixed berries (such as strawberries, blueberries, and raspberries)
- 2 tablespoons granola
- 1 tablespoon honey or maple syrup (optional)
- Fresh mint leaves for garnish (optional)

Instructions:

- In a serving glass or bowl, layer Greek yogurt, mixed berries, and granola.
- Drizzle honey or maple syrup over the top, if desired.
- Garnish with fresh mint leaves for a pop of color and flavor.
- Serve immediately.

Health Benefits:

- This Greek yogurt parfait with berries is a nutritious and satisfying snack option.
- Greek yogurt provides protein and probiotics, which support digestive health.
- Berries are rich in antioxidants and fiber, while granola adds crunch and additional fiber.
- This snack is low in fat and gentle on the gallbladder, making it a great choice for a quick and healthy treat.

Preparation Time: Approximately 5 minutes

2: Hummus and Vegetable Crudité Platter

Ingredients:

- 1/2 cup hummus (store-bought or homemade)

- Assorted vegetables for dipping (such as carrot sticks, cucumber slices, bell pepper strips, and cherry tomatoes)
- Whole-grain crackers or pita bread (optional)
- Lemon wedges for serving (optional)

Instructions:

- Arrange hummus in the center of a serving platter or plate.
- Surround the hummus with assorted vegetable crudité for dipping.
- If desired, add whole-grain crackers or pita bread to the platter for additional crunch.
- Serve with lemon wedges on the side for squeezing over the vegetables, if desired.
- Enjoy!

Health Benefits:

- This hummus and vegetable crudité platter is a nutritious and satisfying snack option.

- Hummus provides plant-based protein and healthy fats, while vegetables offer vitamins, minerals, and fiber.
- Whole-grain crackers or pita bread add complex carbohydrates and additional fiber.

Preparation Time: Approximately 10 minutes

3: Apple Slices with Almond Butter

Ingredients:

- 1 apple, sliced
- 2 tablespoons almond butter
- Cinnamon for sprinkling (optional)

Instructions:

- Slice the apple into wedges or rounds.
- Spread almond butter onto each apple slice.
- Sprinkle with cinnamon, if desired.
- Serve immediately.

Health Benefits:

- This snack of apple slices with almond butter is a simple and nutritious option.

- Apples are rich in fiber and antioxidants, while almond butter provides healthy fats and protein.
- The combination of sweet apple and creamy almond butter makes for a satisfying and gallbladder-friendly snack.

Preparation Time: Approximately 5 minutes

4: Cottage Cheese and Pineapple Kabobs

Ingredients:

- 1 cup cottage cheese
- 1 cup pineapple chunks (fresh or canned)
- Bamboo skewers

Instructions:

- Thread pineapple chunks and cottage cheese onto bamboo skewers, alternating between the two.
- Repeat until all ingredients are used.
- Serve immediately.

Health Benefits:

- This snack of cottage cheese and pineapple kabobs is a refreshing and protein-packed option.

- Cottage cheese is a good source of protein and calcium, while pineapple provides vitamins, minerals, and digestive enzymes. Enjoying them together on skewers makes for a fun and satisfying snack that's gentle on the gallbladder.

Preparation Time: Approximately 10 minutes

5: Avocado Toast with Tomato

Ingredients:

- 2 slices whole-grain bread
- 1 ripe avocado
- 1 small tomato, sliced
- Salt and pepper to taste
- Red pepper flakes for garnish (optional)
- Fresh cilantro or basil for garnish (optional)

Instructions:

- Toast the slices of whole-grain bread until golden brown.
- While the bread is toasting, mash the ripe avocado in a bowl with a fork until smooth.

- Spread mashed avocado evenly onto each slice of toasted bread.
- Top the avocado toast with sliced tomatoes.
- Season with salt and pepper to taste.
- Garnish with red pepper flakes, fresh cilantro, or basil, if desired.
- Serve immediately.

Health Benefits:

- This avocado toast with tomato is a delicious and nutritious snack option.
- Avocado provides healthy fats, vitamins, and minerals, while whole-grain bread offers fiber and complex carbohydrates.
- Tomatoes add vitamins and antioxidants.

Preparation Time: Approximately 10 minutes

6: Rice Cake with Almond Butter and Banana

Ingredients:

- 1 rice cake
- 1 tablespoon almond butter
- 1/2 banana, sliced

- Honey for drizzling (optional)
- Chia seeds for garnish (optional)

Instructions:

- Spread almond butter evenly onto the rice cake.
- Top the almond butter with sliced banana.
- Drizzle with honey, if desired.
- Sprinkle with chia seeds for added texture and nutrition, if desired.
- Serve immediately.

Health Benefits:

- This rice cake with almond butter and banana is a quick and satisfying snack option.
- Rice cakes are low in calories and fat, while almond butter provides healthy fats and protein.
- Bananas are rich in potassium and fiber.

Preparation Time: Approximately 5 minutes

7: Veggie Sticks with Yogurt Dip

Ingredients:

- Assorted vegetable sticks (carrots, cucumber, bell peppers, celery)
- 1/2 cup Greek yogurt
- 1 tablespoon lemon juice
- 1 teaspoon dried dill
- Salt and pepper to taste

Instructions:

- Wash and cut assorted vegetables into sticks.
- In a small bowl, mix Greek yogurt, lemon juice, dried dill, salt, and pepper until well combined.
- Serve the vegetable sticks with the yogurt dip on the side.
- Enjoy!

Health Benefits:

- This snack is packed with nutrients from the assorted vegetables and Greek yogurt dip.

- Vegetables provide vitamins, minerals, and fiber, while Greek yogurt offers protein and probiotics for gut health.

Preparation Time: Approximately 10 minutes

8: Almond and Berry Smoothie

Ingredients:

- 1/2 cup frozen mixed berries (such as strawberries, blueberries, raspberries)
- 1 ripe banana
- 1 tablespoon almond butter
- 1 cup almond milk (or any milk of your choice)
- 1 tablespoon honey or maple syrup (optional)
- Ice cubes (optional)

Instructions:

- Place frozen mixed berries, ripe banana, almond butter, almond milk, and honey or maple syrup (if using) in a blender.
- Blend until smooth and creamy.
- If desired, add ice cubes to the blender and blend again until smooth.

- Pour the smoothie into a glass and serve immediately.

Health Benefits:

- This almond and berry smoothie is a delicious and nutritious snack option.
- Berries are packed with antioxidants and fiber, while almond butter provides healthy fats and protein. Bananas add natural sweetness and potassium.

Preparation Time: Approximately 5 minutes

9: Baked Sweet Potato Chips

Ingredients:

- 1 large sweet potato
- 1 tablespoon olive oil
- Salt and pepper to taste
- Optional: paprika, garlic powder, or other seasonings of choice

Instructions:

- Preheat the oven to 375°F (190°C) and line a baking sheet with parchment paper.

- Wash and dry the sweet potato, then thinly slice it into rounds using a sharp knife or mandoline slicer.
- In a large bowl, toss the sweet potato slices with olive oil, salt, pepper, and any additional seasonings of choice until evenly coated.
- Arrange the sweet potato slices in a single layer on the prepared baking sheet.
- Bake in the preheated oven for 15-20 minutes, flipping halfway through, or until the chips are crispy and golden brown.
- Remove from the oven and let cool slightly before serving.
- Enjoy these baked sweet potato chips as a healthy and satisfying snack!

Health Benefits:

- Sweet potatoes are rich in fiber, vitamins, and minerals, making them a nutritious alternative to regular potato chips.
- Baking the sweet potato slices with olive oil instead of frying reduces the fat content, making this snack gentle on the gallbladder.

Preparation Time: Approximately 25 minutes

10: Cottage Cheese and Fruit Bowl

Ingredients:

- 1/2 cup cottage cheese
- 1/2 cup mixed fresh fruit (such as berries, pineapple, kiwi, or mango)
- 1 tablespoon chopped nuts (such as almonds, walnuts, or pecans)
- Optional: honey or maple syrup for drizzling

Instructions:

- Spoon the cottage cheese into a bowl.
- Top with mixed fresh fruit and chopped nuts.
- Drizzle with honey or maple syrup if desired.
- Serve immediately and enjoy this simple and satisfying snack!

Health Benefits:

- Cottage cheese is a good source of protein and calcium, while fresh fruit provides vitamins, minerals, and antioxidants.

- Nuts add healthy fats and crunch.
- This cottage cheese and fruit bowl is a balanced and nutritious snack that's gentle on the gallbladder and easy to prepare. Customize it with your favorite fruits and nuts for variety.

Preparation Time: Approximately 5 minutes

CONCLUSION

Adopting a gallbladder diet for beginners offers not only relief from discomfort but also promotes overall digestive health and well-being.

By incorporating nutrient-rich foods, such as lean proteins, fruits, vegetables, whole grains, and healthy fats, individuals can support gallbladder function while enjoying delicious and satisfying meals and snacks.

Furthermore, following the guidelines of a gallbladder diet can help prevent the formation of gallstones and alleviate symptoms associated with gallbladder issues, such as bloating, indigestion, and abdominal pain. With easy-to-follow recipes and simple yet effective dietary adjustments, beginners can embark on a journey towards improved digestive health and quality of life.

Remember, always consult with a healthcare professional or registered dietitian before making significant changes to your diet, especially if you have existing medical conditions or concerns. By taking proactive steps to prioritize gallbladder health through diet, beginners can pave the way for long-term wellness and vitality.
Start today and discover the transformative benefits of a gallbladder-friendly lifestyle.

www.ingramcontent.com/pod-product-compliance
Lightning Source LLC
Chambersburg PA
CBHW050234230526
45470CB00005B/1953